Don't forget to wash your Kitty-Cat

By M.S.Woodley

This book is dedicated to my mother Dianna Woodley-Sapp

For daring to think outside the box; Thank you for not teaching your four girls that the "stork" is responsible for bringing new bundles of joy to people and most of all Thank you for making sure that we all washed our Kitty-Cats!

Love your daughter,

M.S. Woodley

Dedication page#2

To my awesome siblings Kim, Isis, and Starkima.

I dedicate this page to you all for making my life so colorful and I am so unbelievably grateful for having each and every one of you for a sibling plus... createspace.com wants me to have twenty four pages in order to upload my book and I was three pages short.

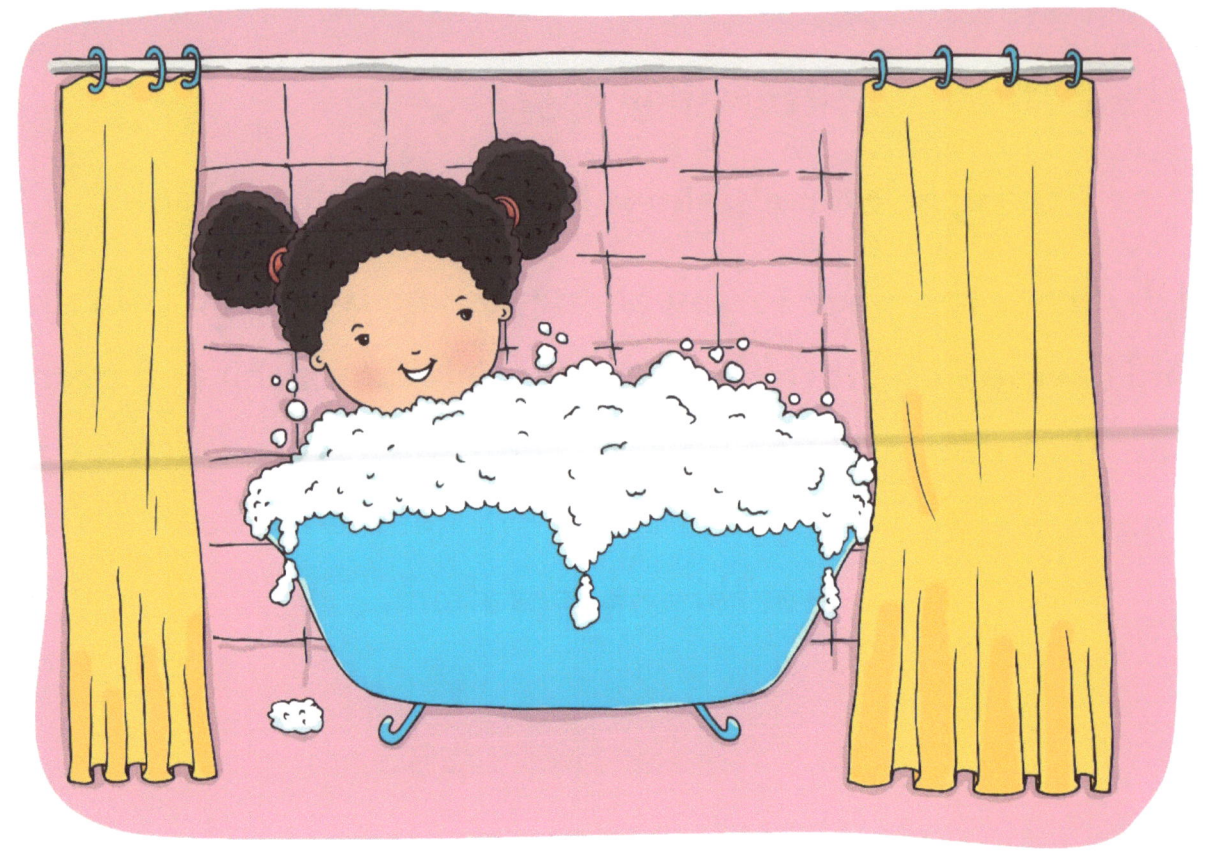

When I take
a bath,

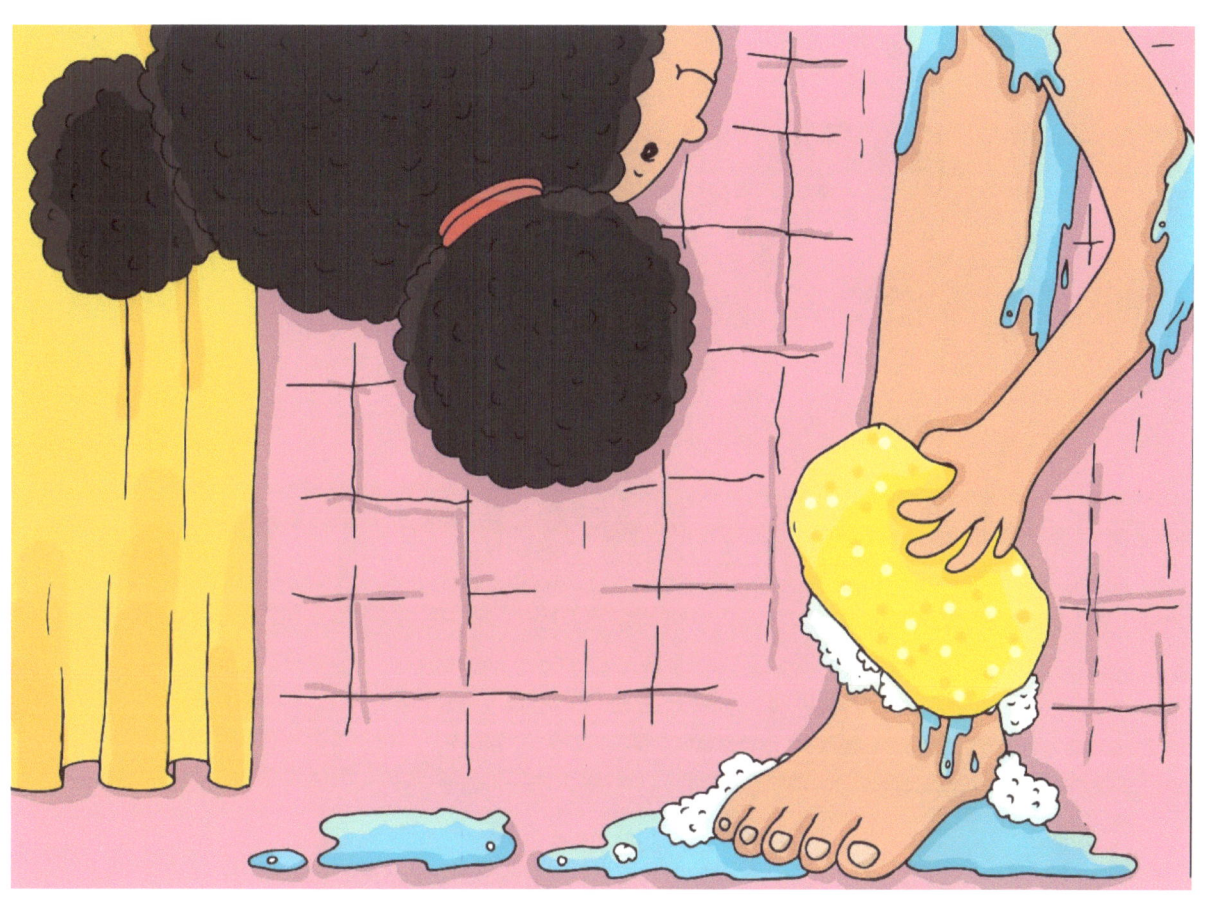

Or just wash up...

Mommy says,

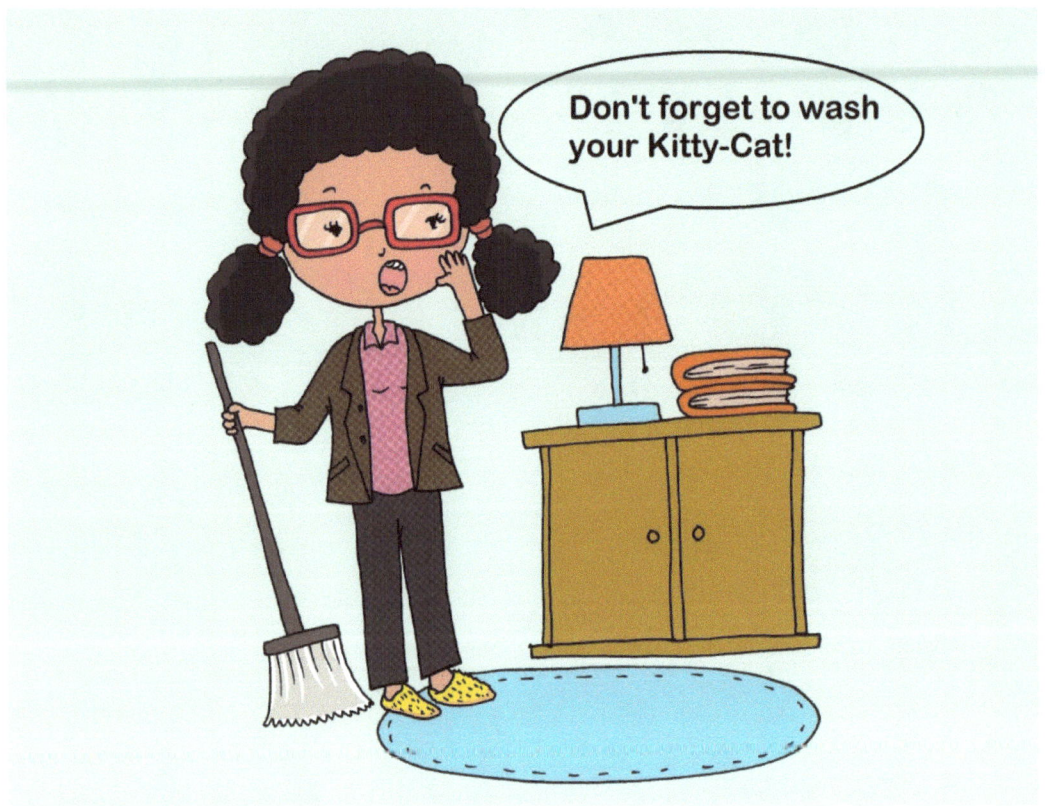

Then I say,

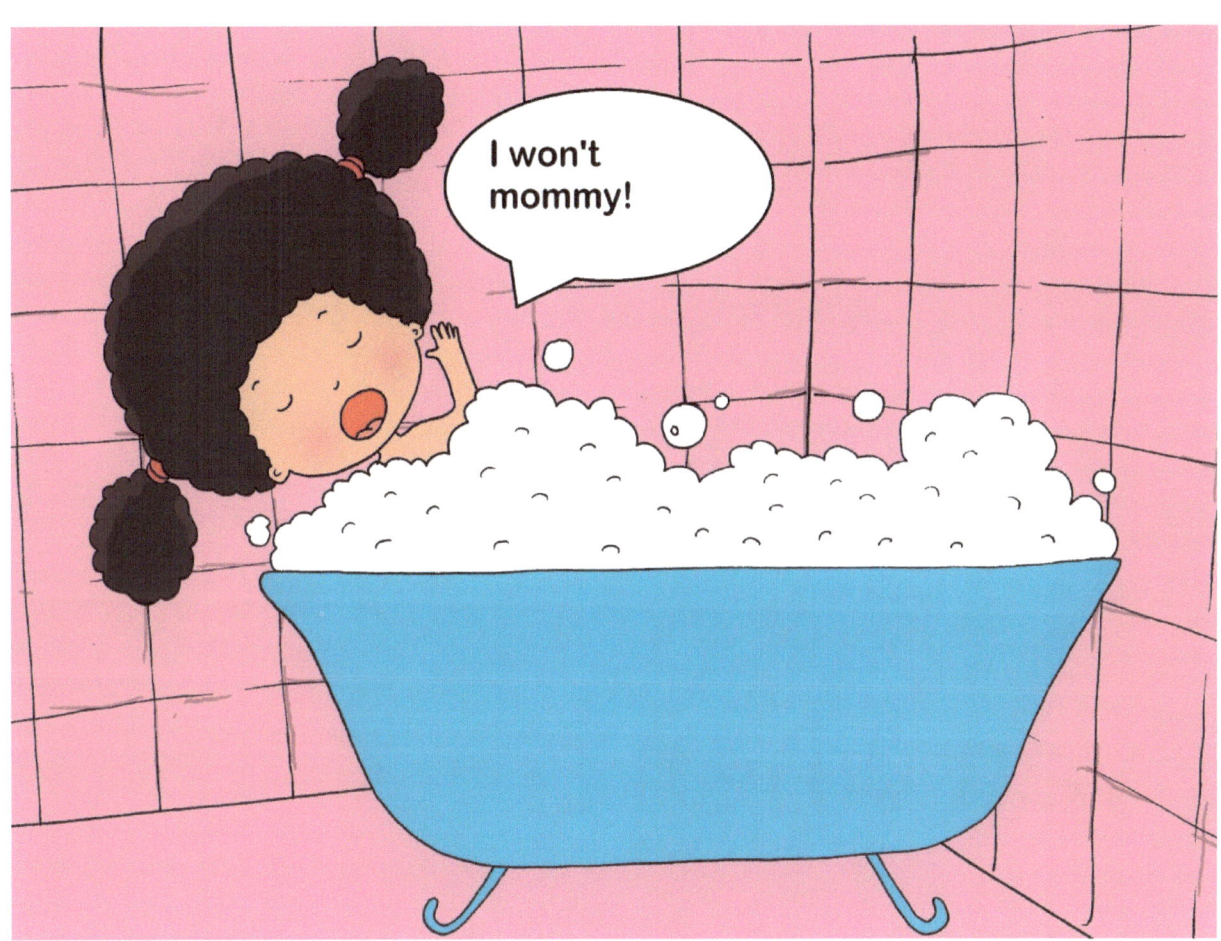

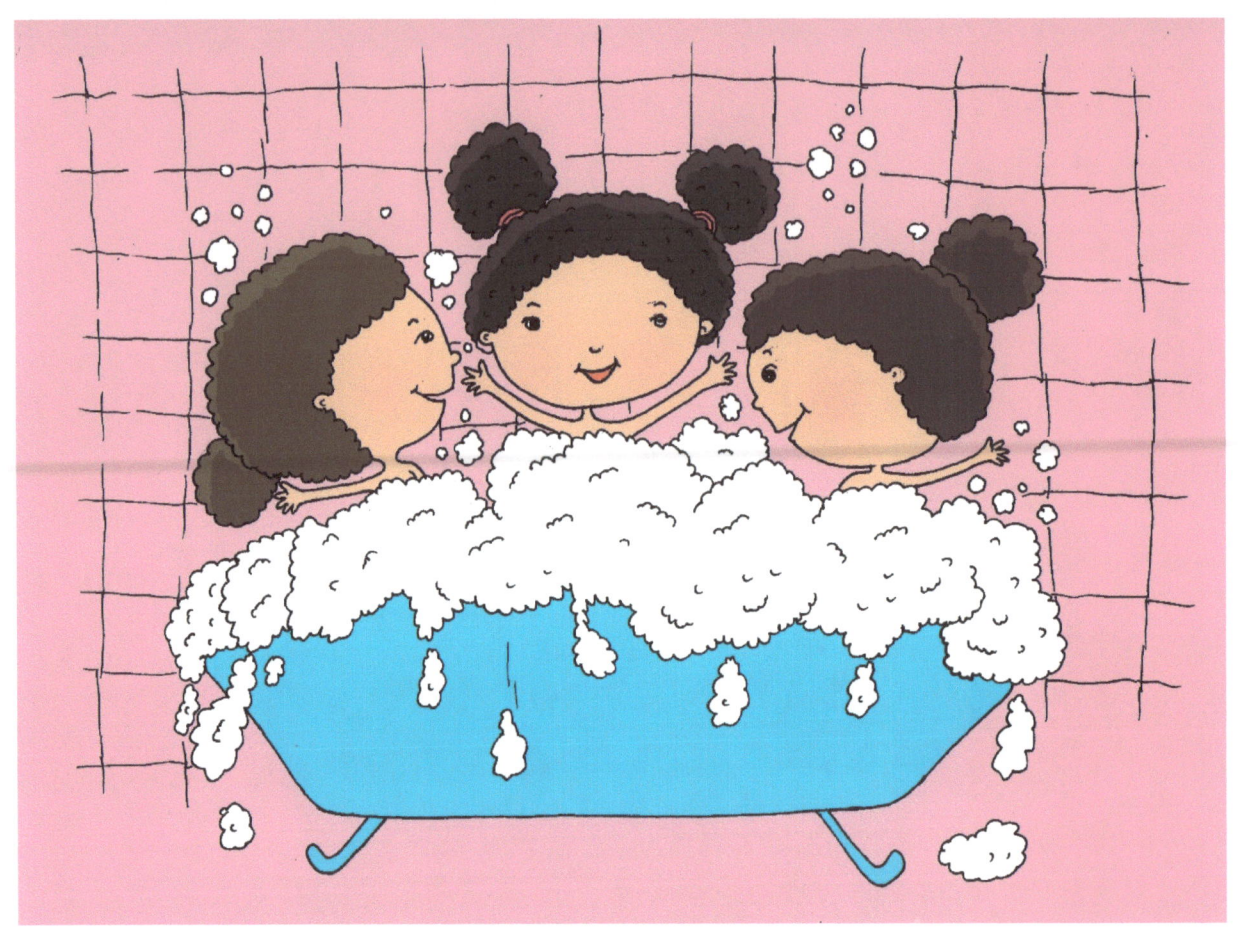

Even when
  I take a bath with
my sisters,

Mommy still says,

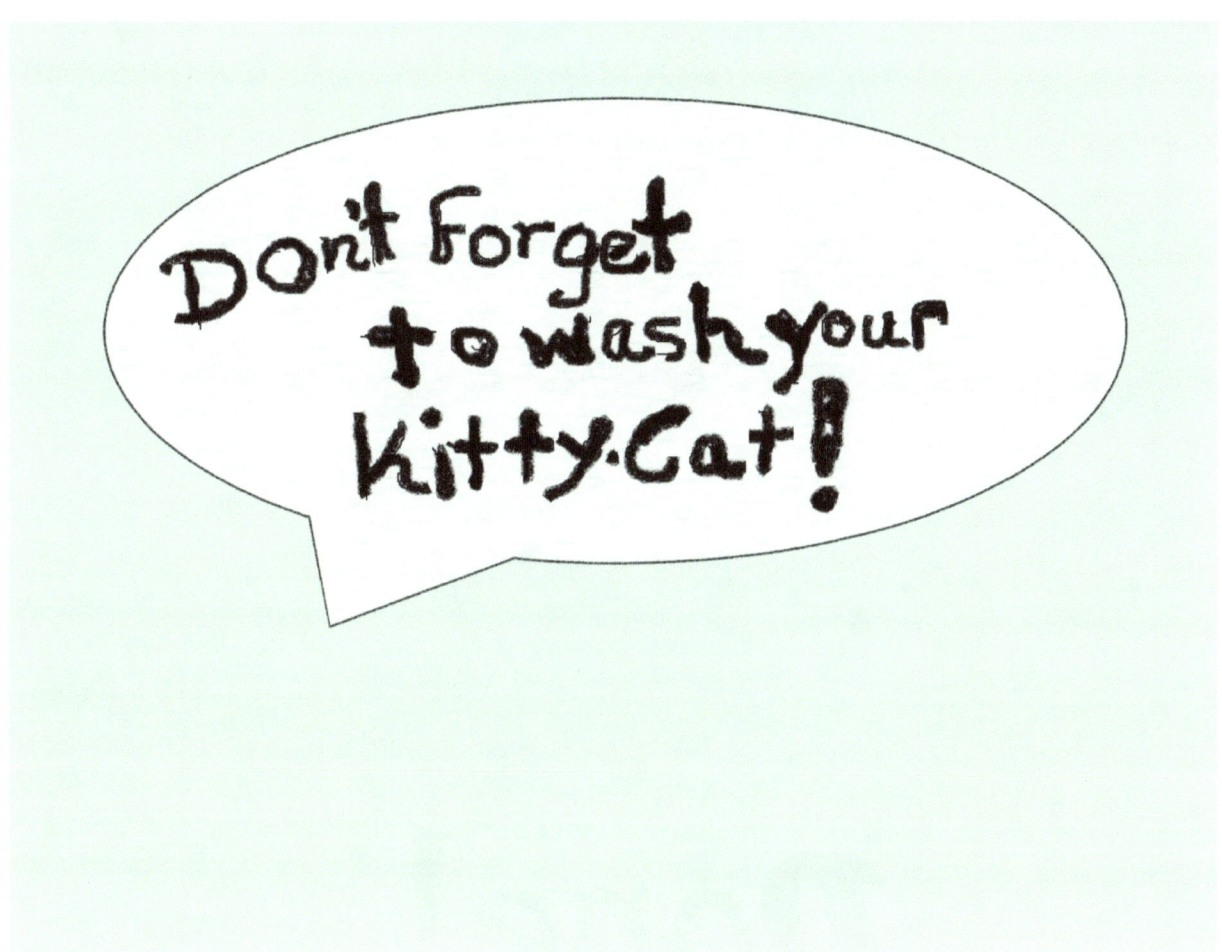

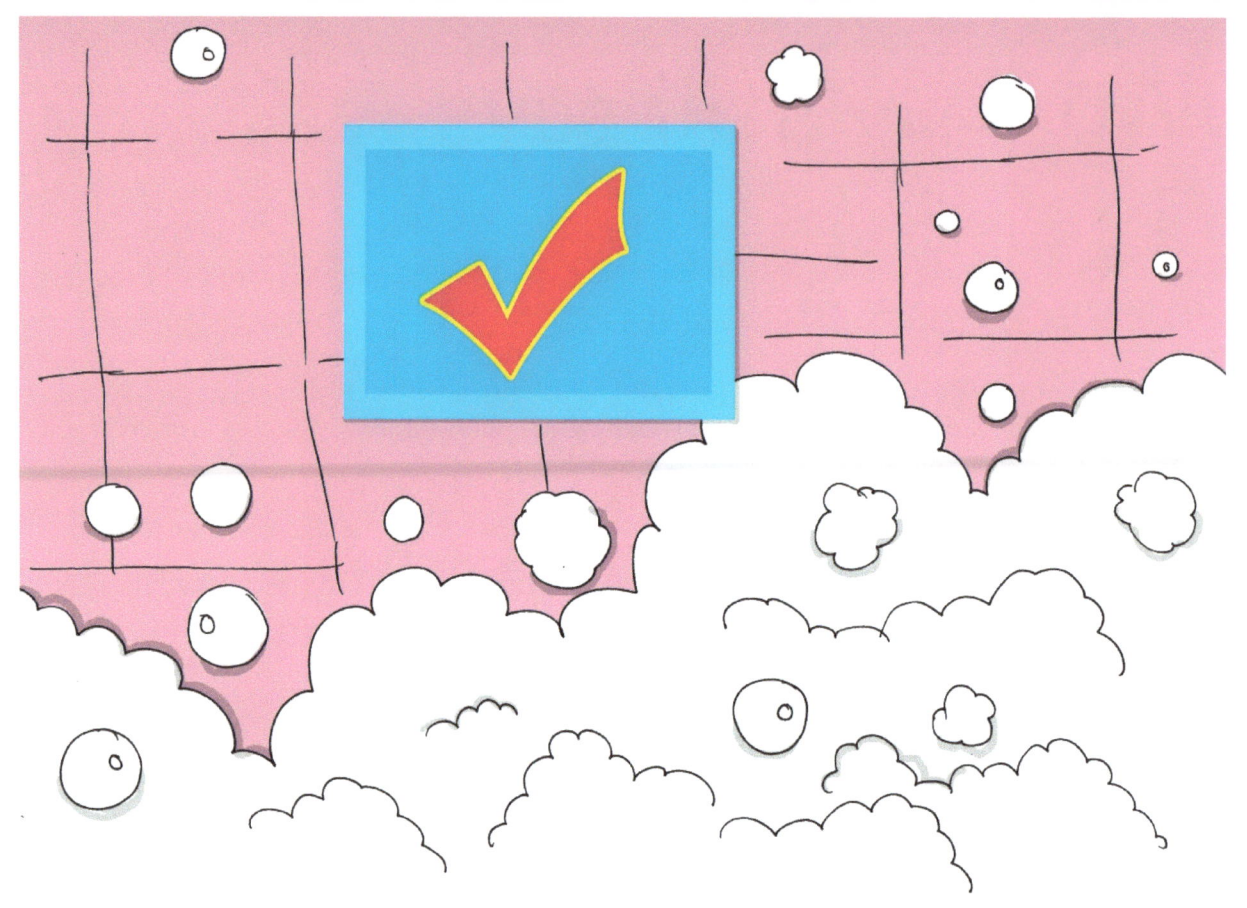

Done!

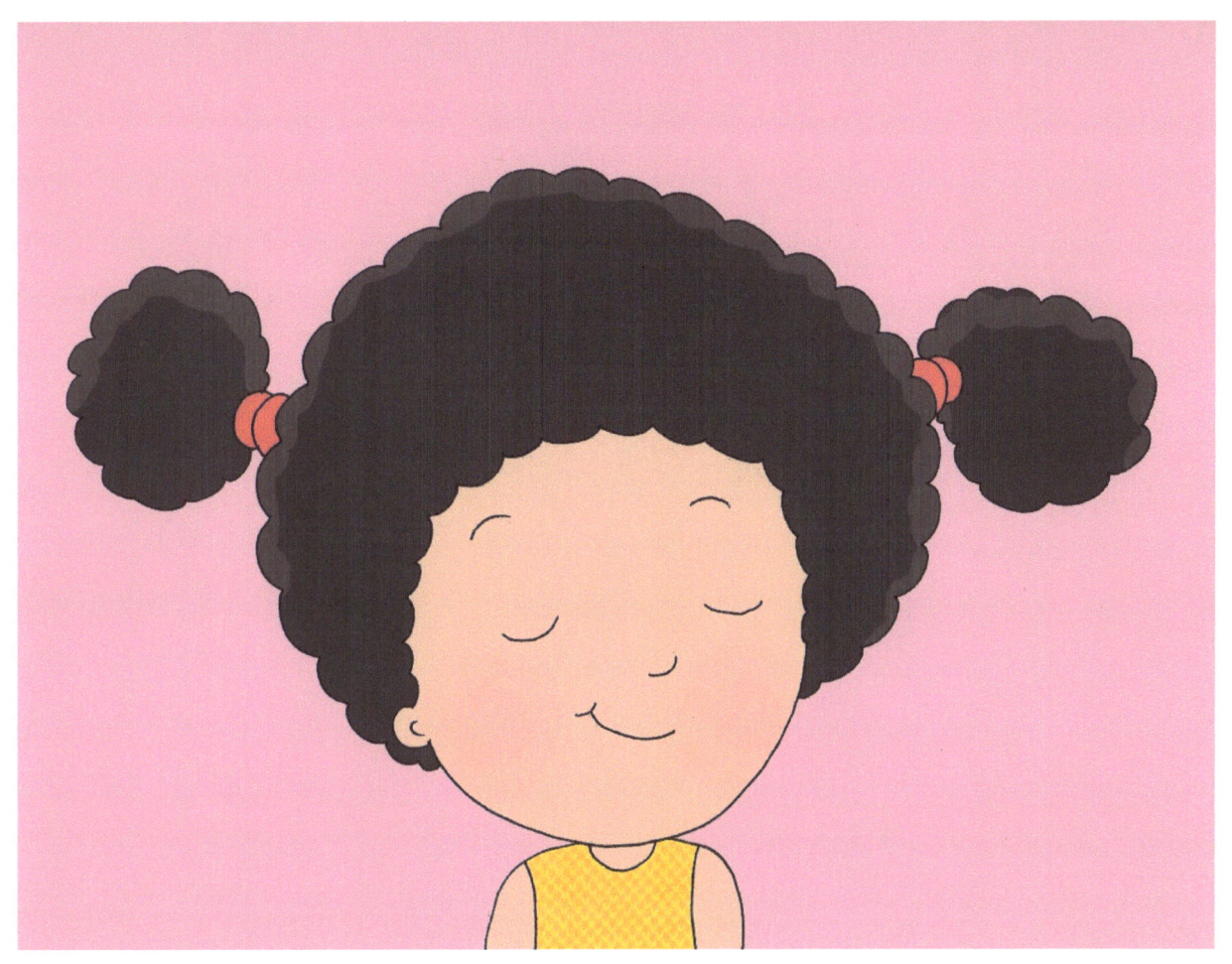

I am very proud of myself for being able to wash my own Kitty-Cat.

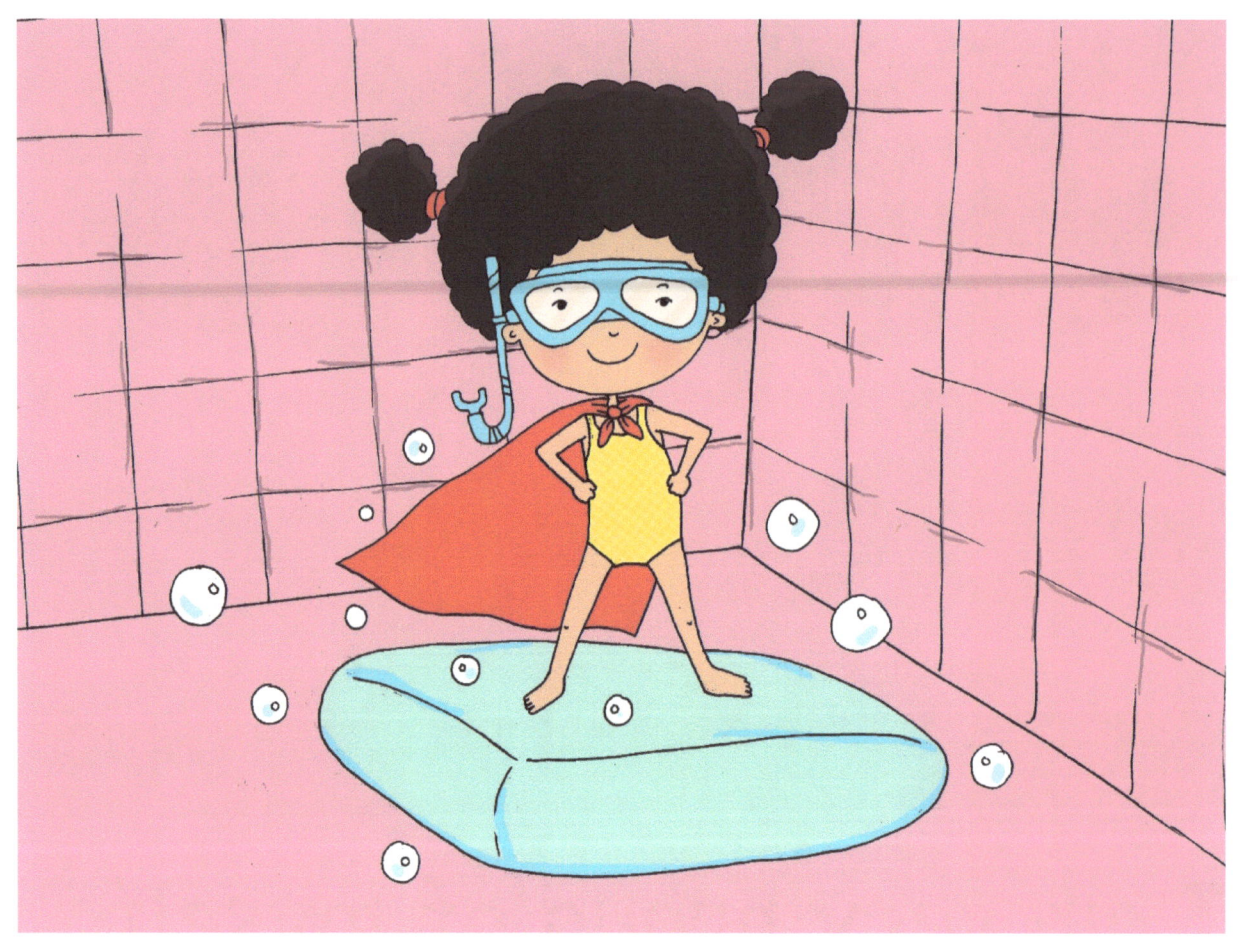

Very, very Proud...

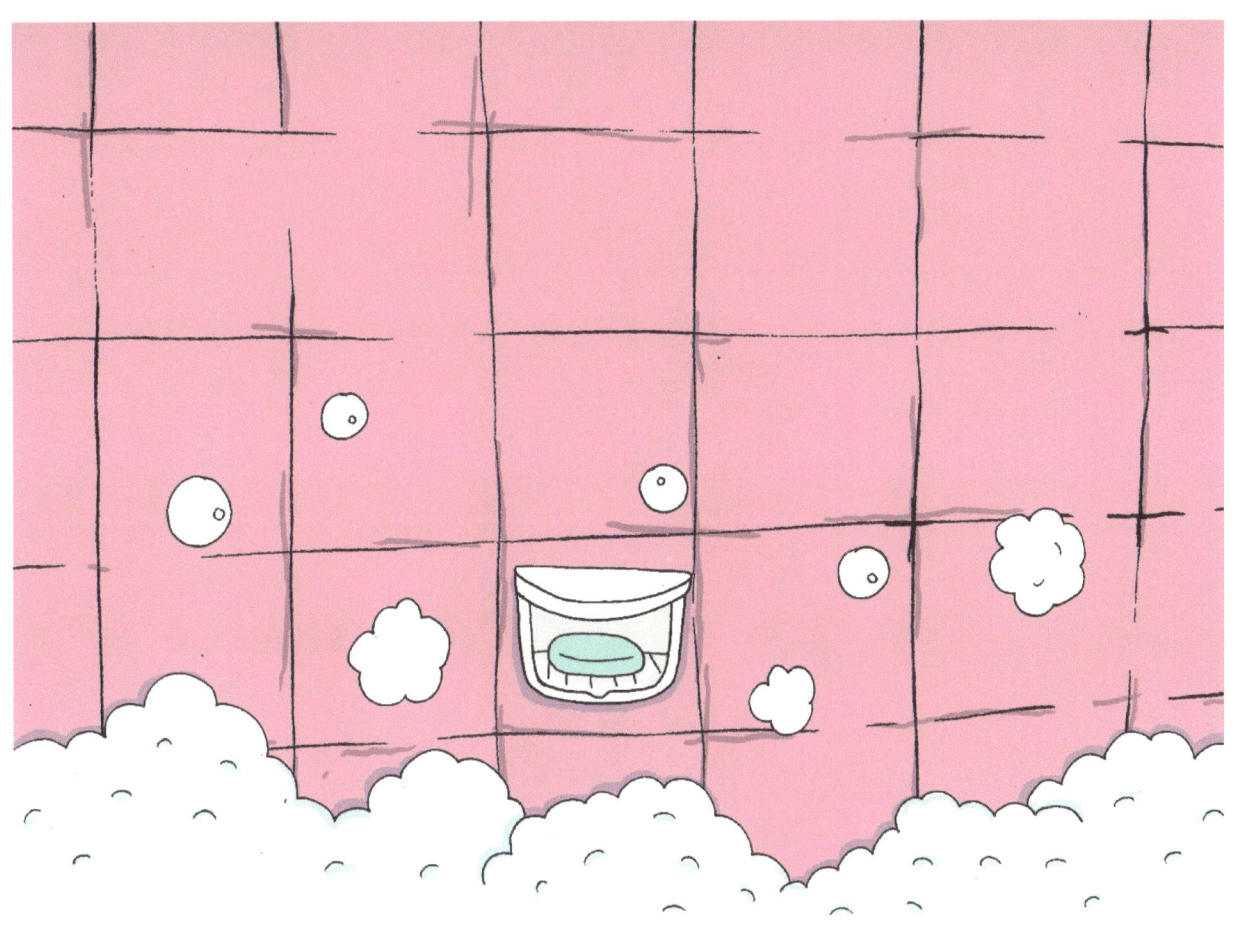

But never use too much
SOAP!

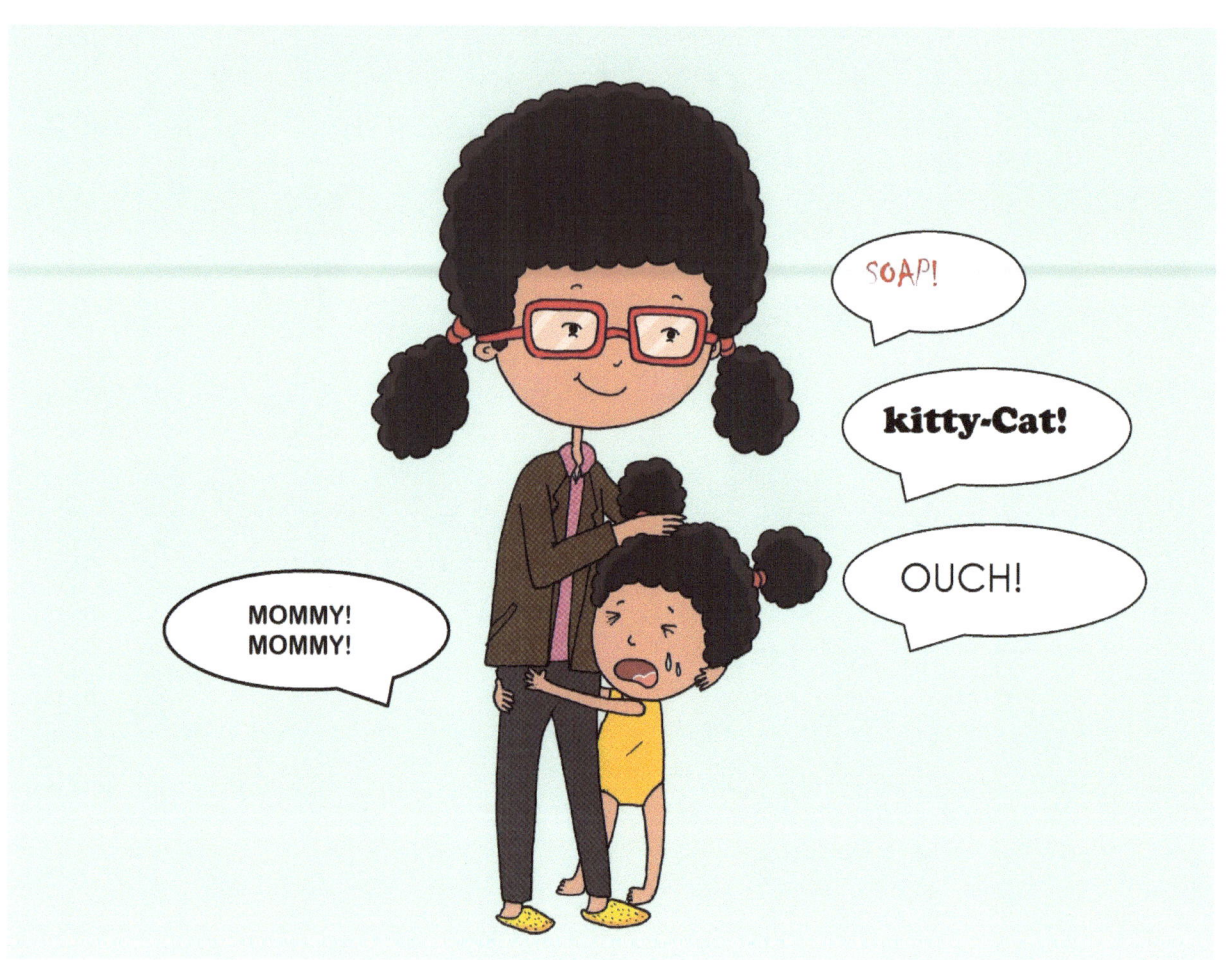

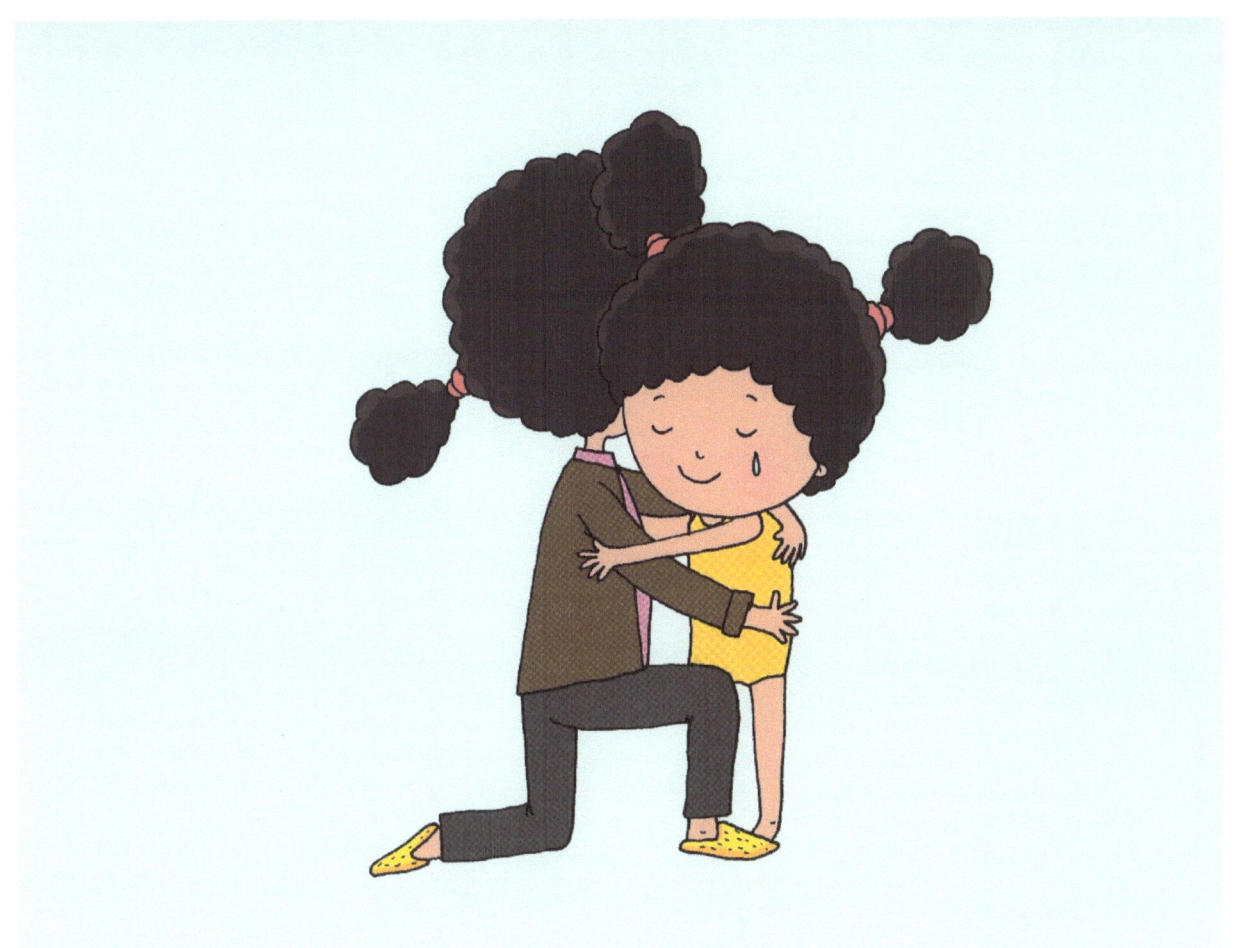

Mommy's hugs and kisses **ALWAYS** make me feel better.

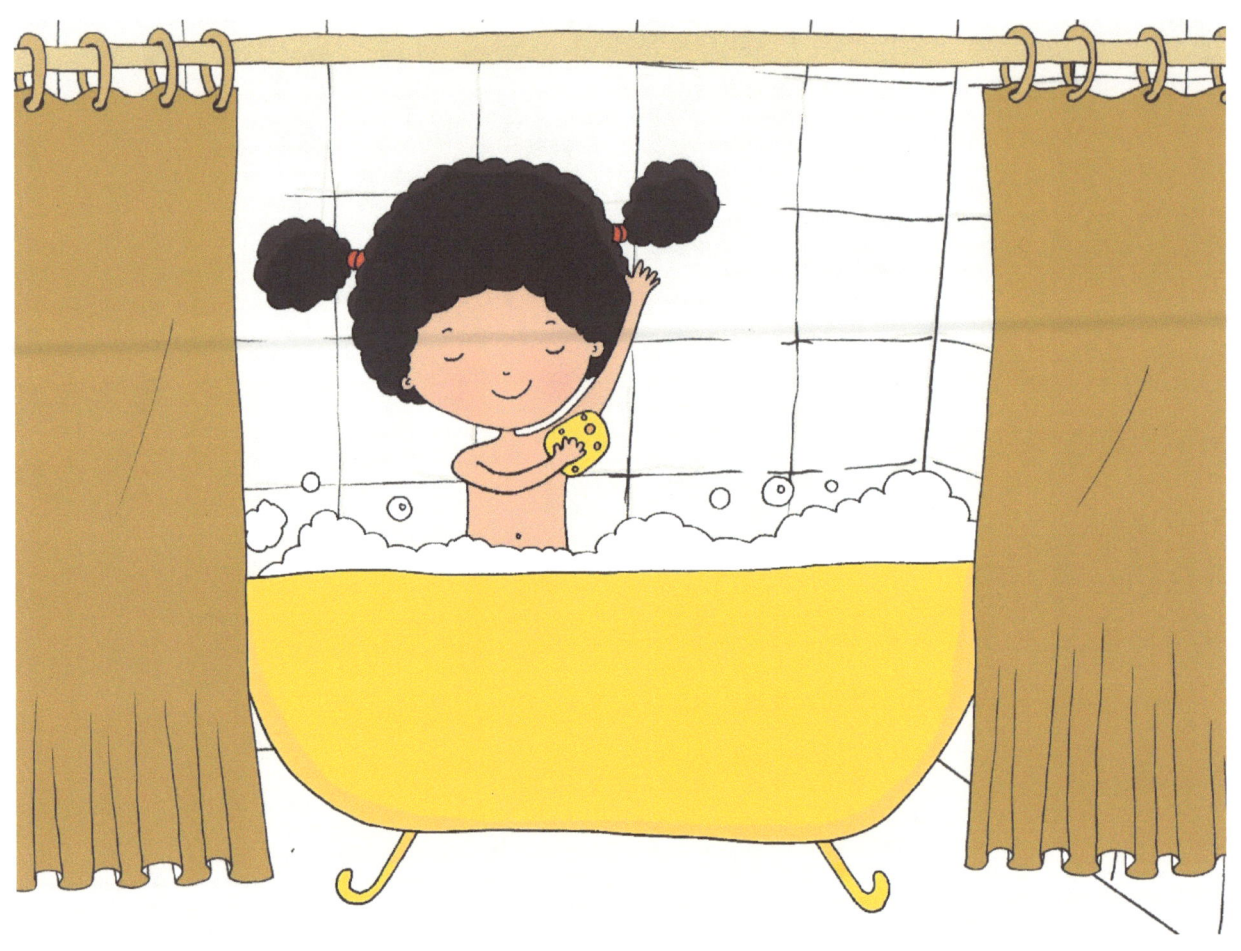

And when I take a bath
at grandma's house, even
grandma says,

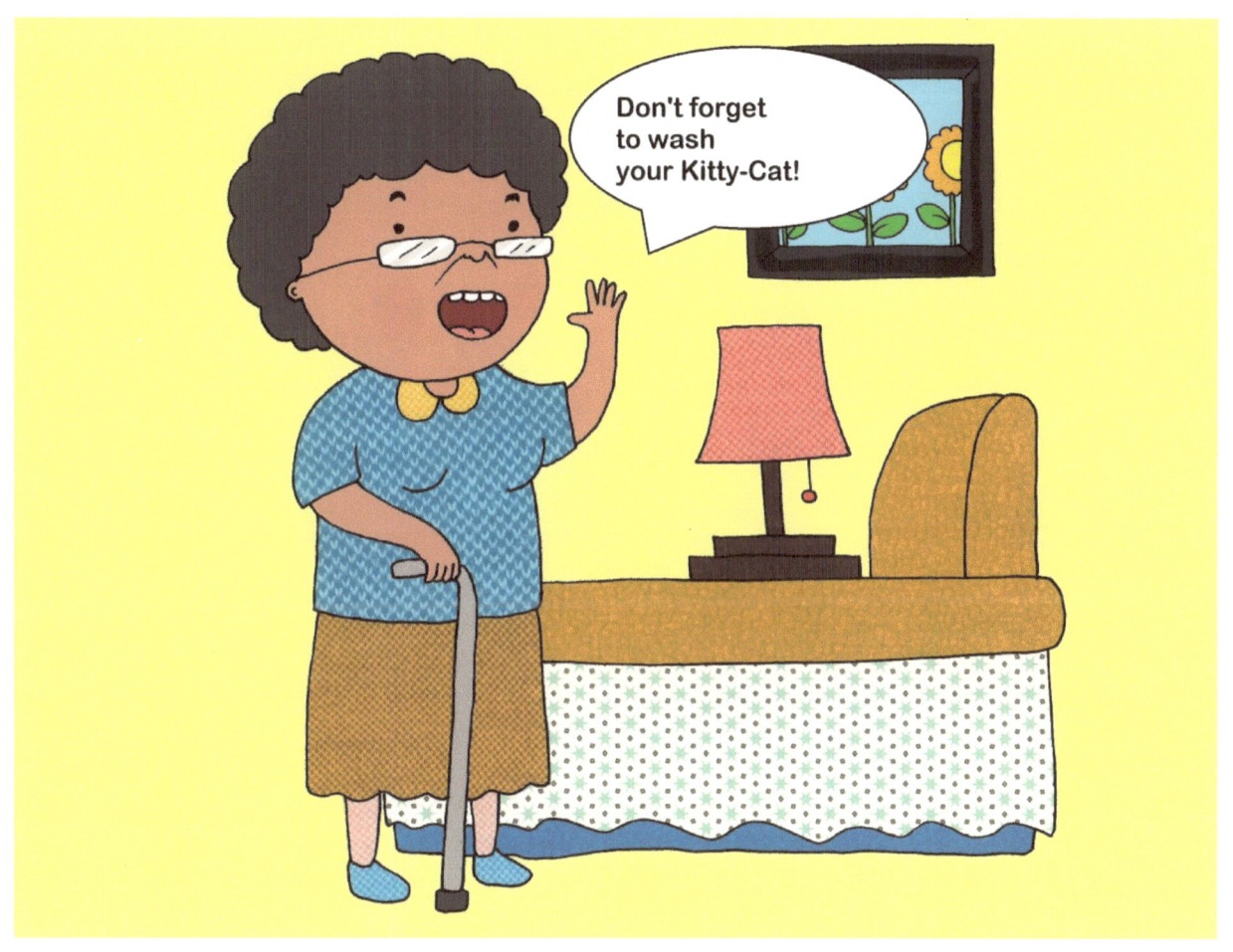

"Okay Grandma, I won't!"

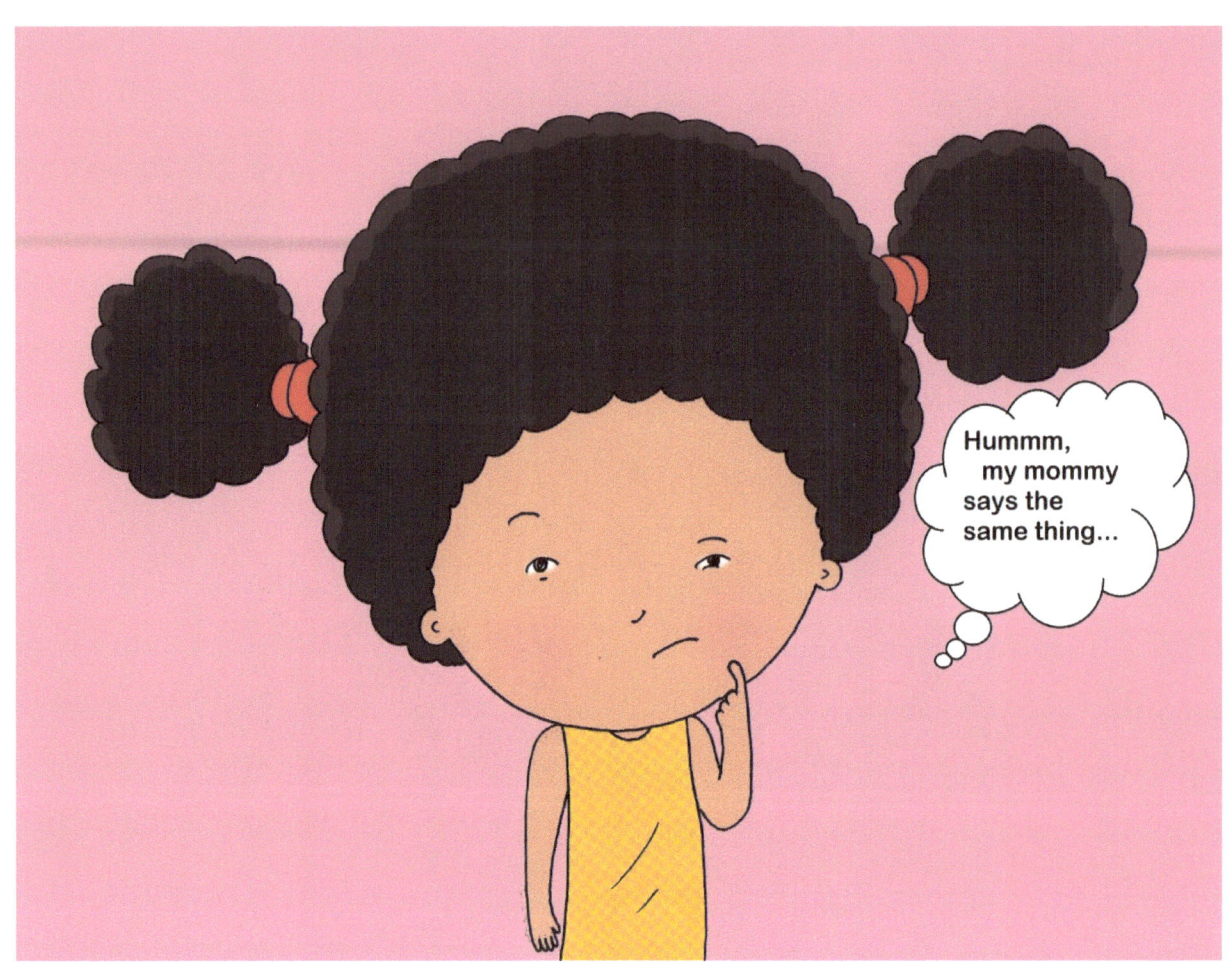

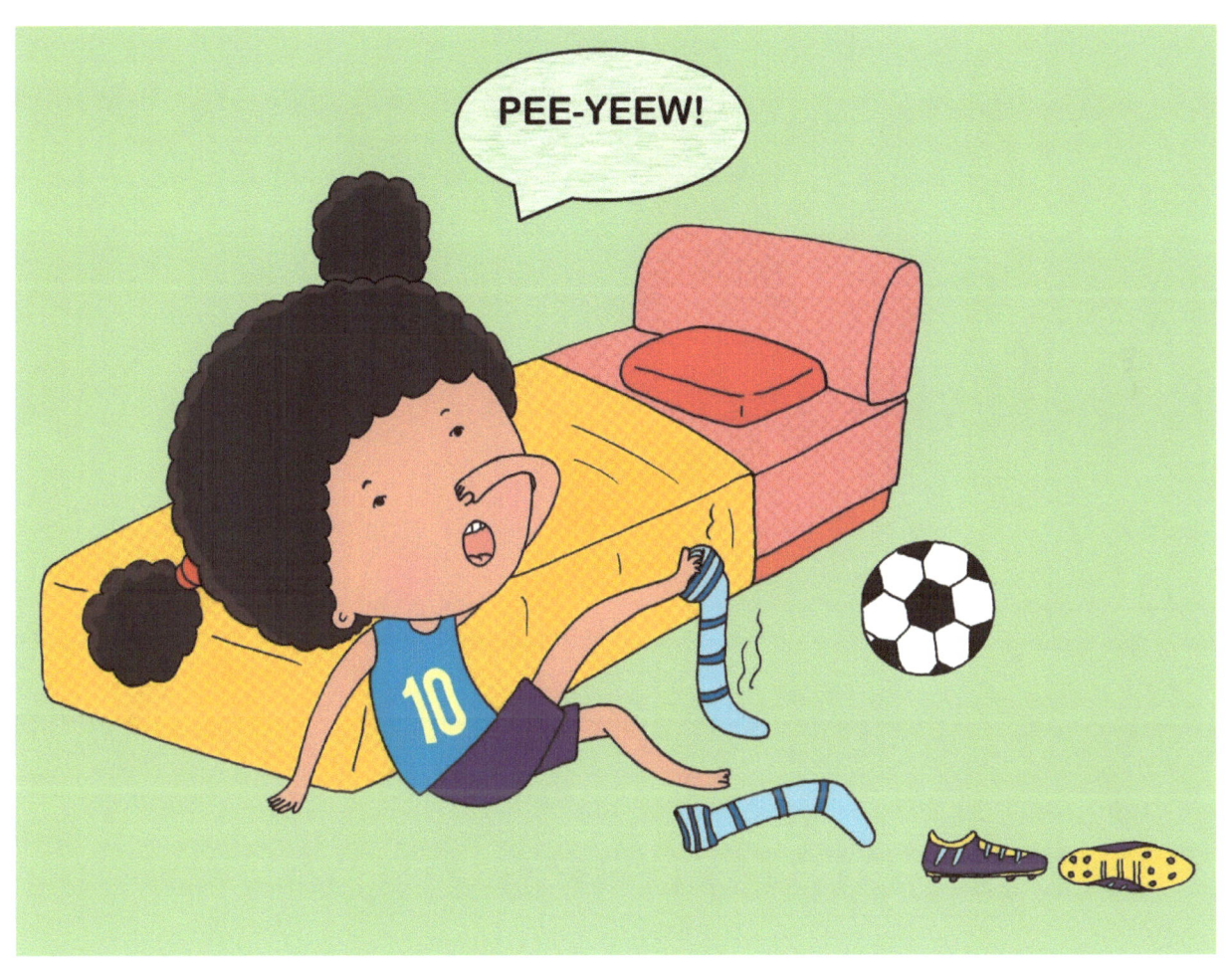

Although I might forget to wash my smelly socks.

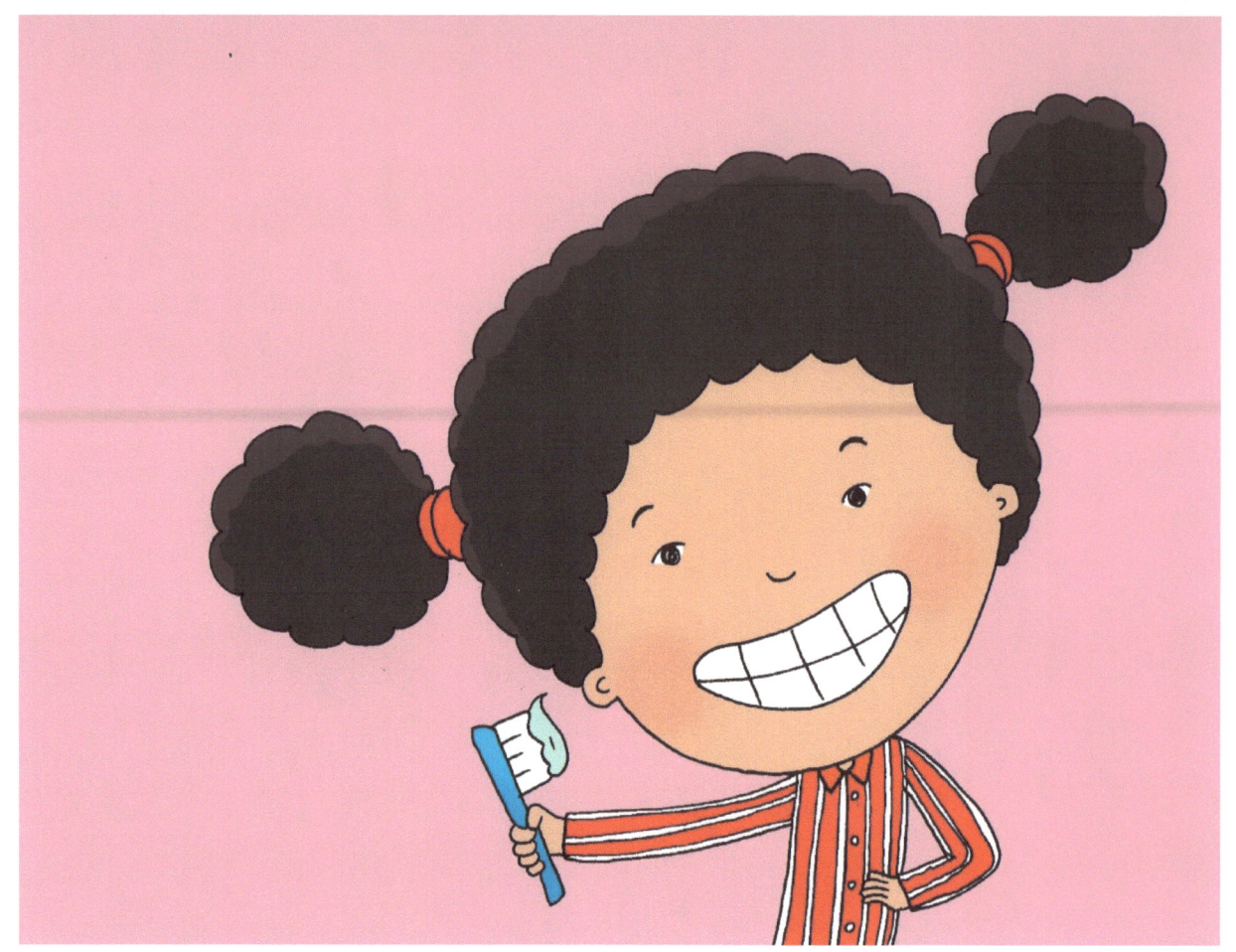

And I sometimes may forget to brush my teeth at night...oops!

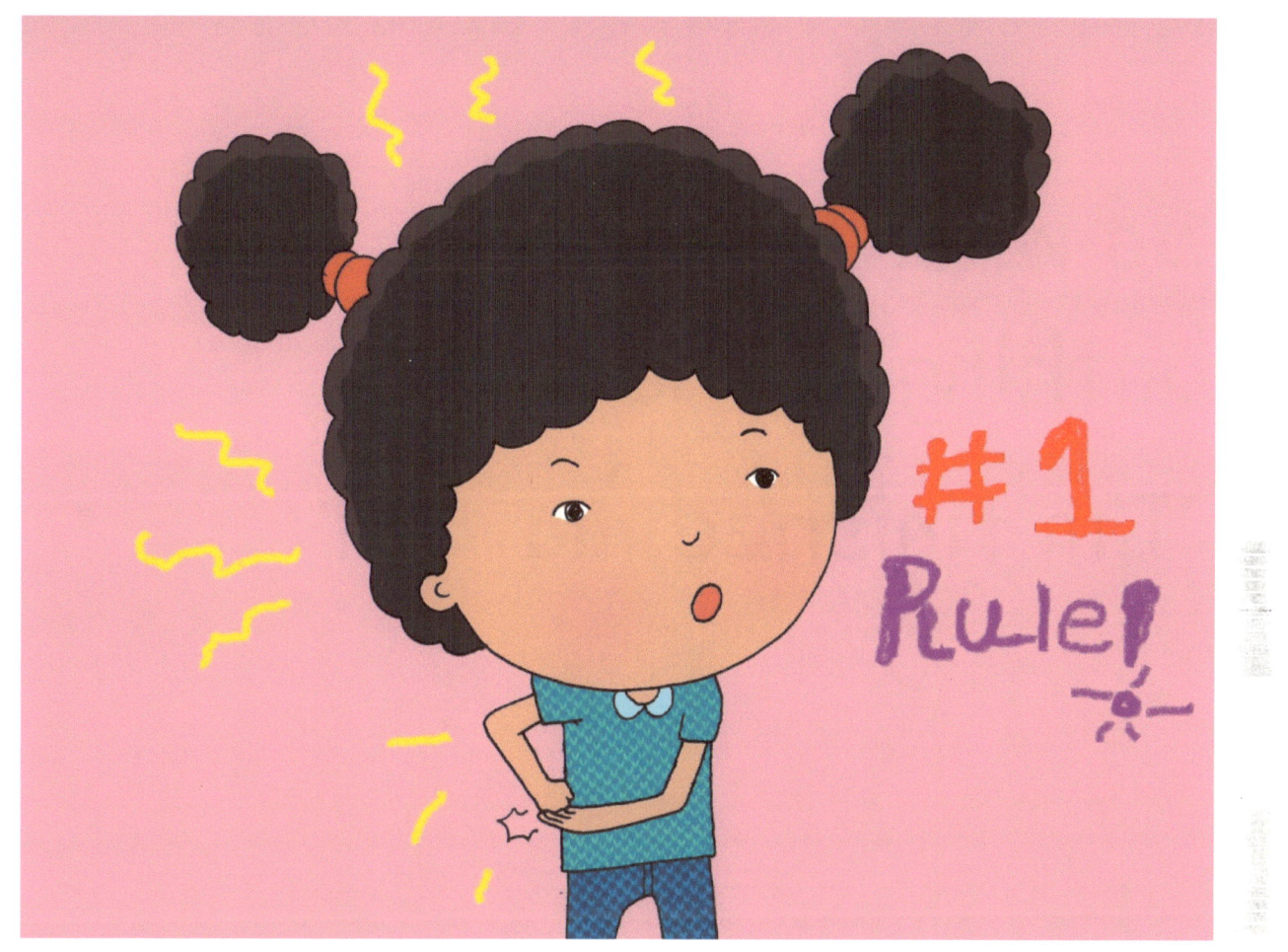

But I will never-ever,

Ever-never, forget to

wash my kitty-Cat.

So when I finish bathing, I shout out,

"I'm finished mommy!"

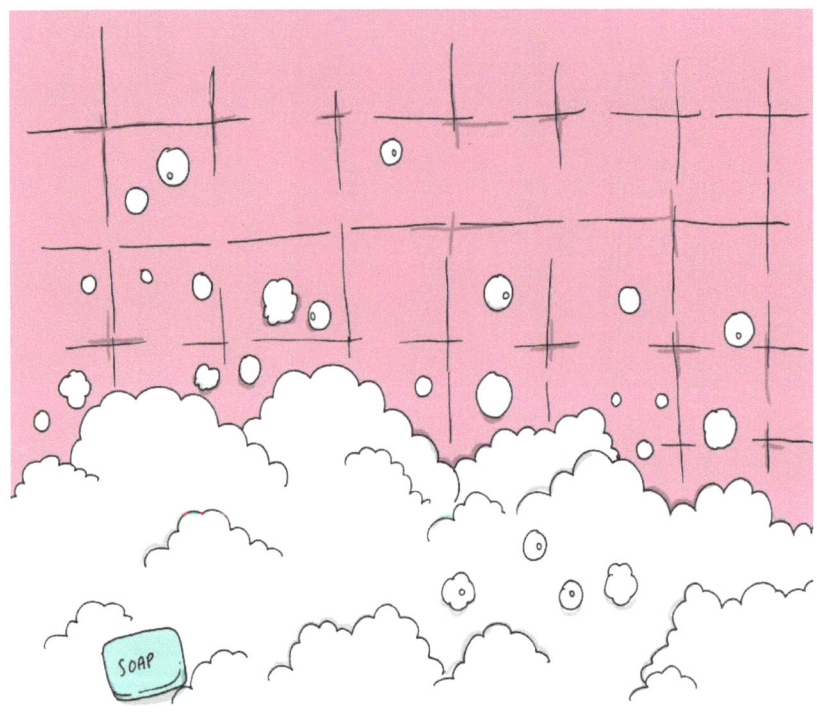

And mommy says,

"Good Job Sweetie, now get ready for bed...!"

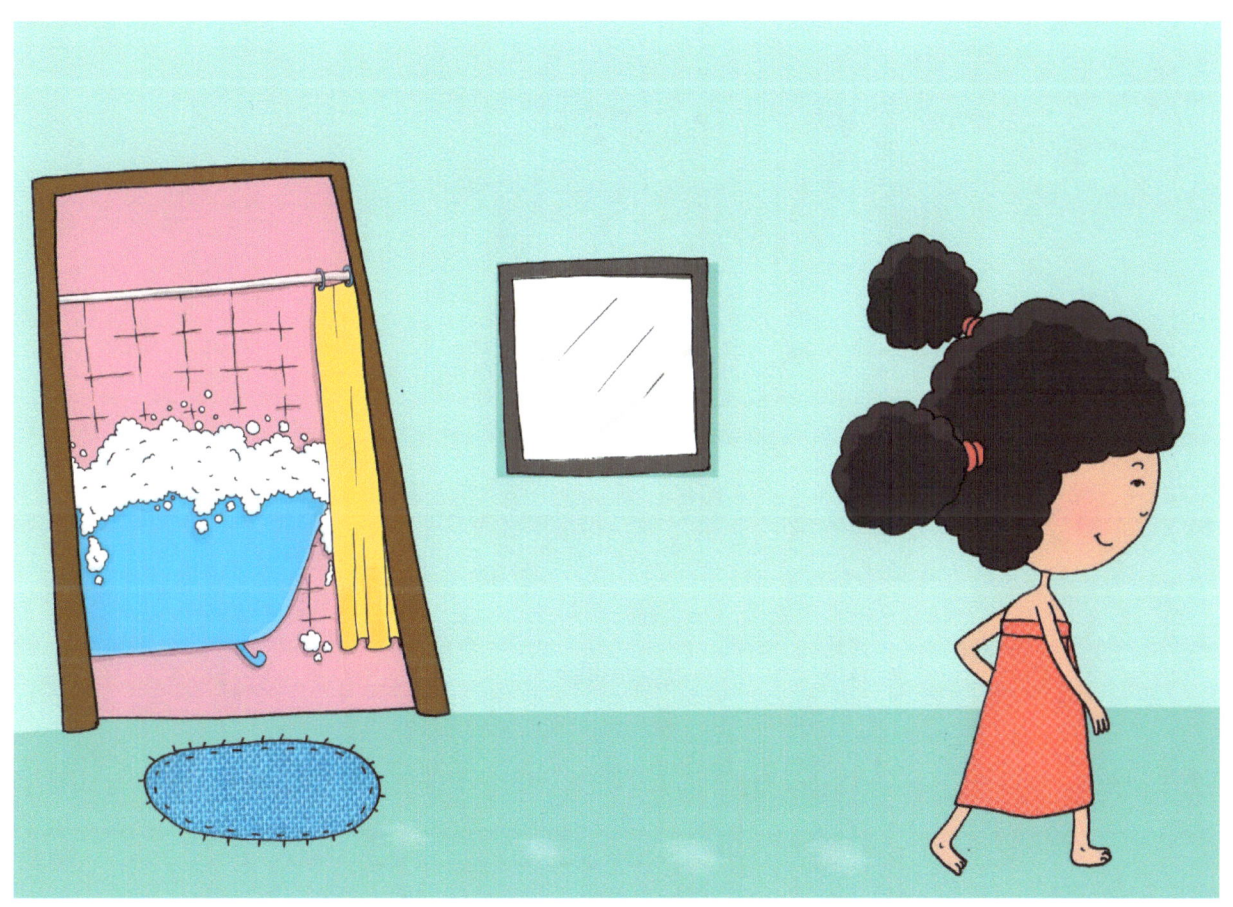

So off to bed I go...

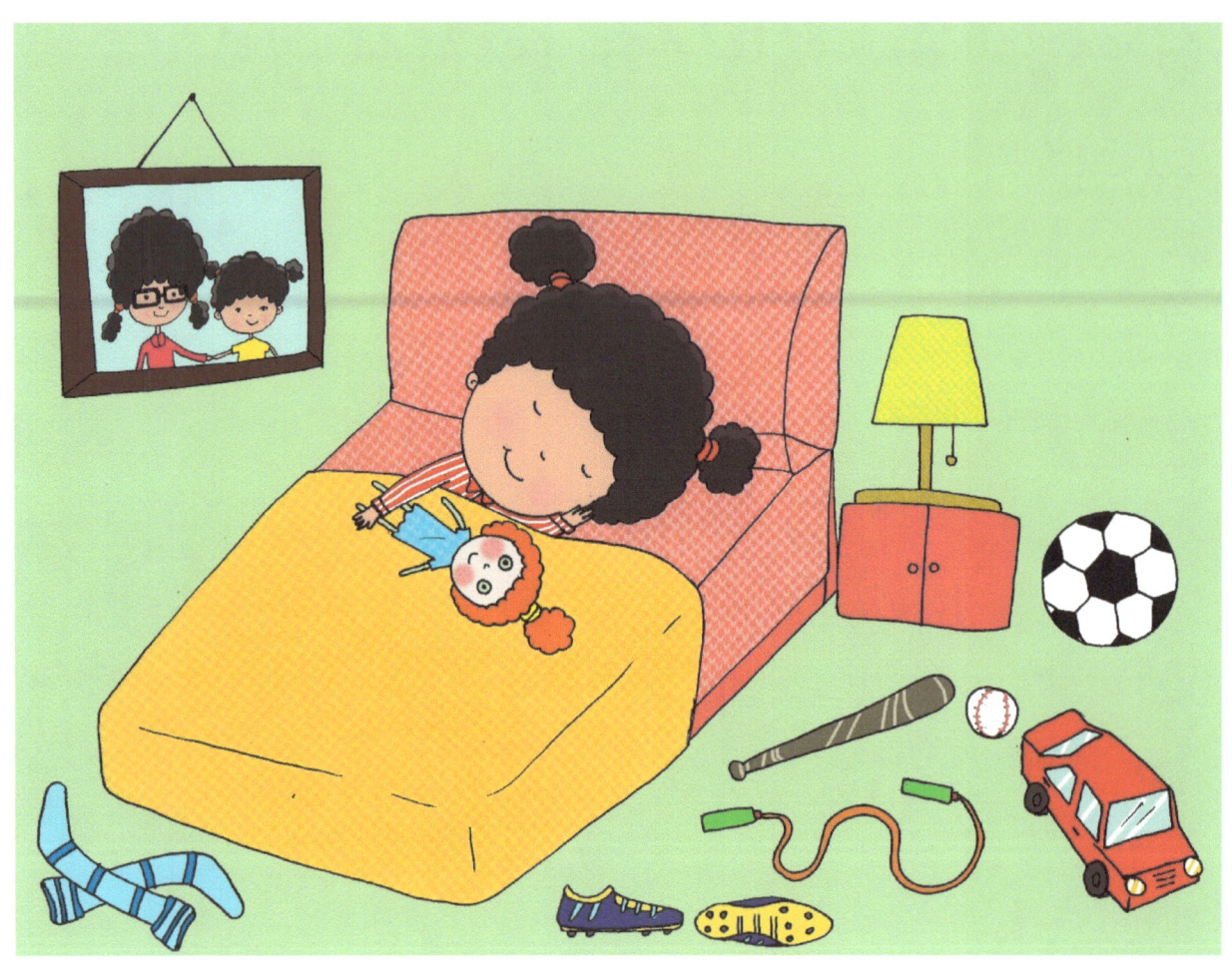

The End...

SPECIAL THANKS

SPUFFS-illustrator

fiverr.com

Adia Stuart Editor

Createspace.com

And to all my friends and family...!

Author M.S. Woodley is a self-proclaimed STORY MANIFESTATOR-ATOR.

She resides in Brooklyn New York with her 5 year old son and his pet goldfish named … Ms.Gold fish.

Contact info mswoodleyauthor@gmail.com

www.ingramcontent.com/pod-product-compliance
Lightning Source LLC
Chambersburg PA
CBHW060817290526
45792CB00005BB/1691

9781500550516